THE ESSEN

CW01501936

HERBALISM

AND

NATURAL REMEDIES

29 FORMULAS FOR COMBINING HERBS INTO
HEALING RECIPES

Author:

KELSEY C. HARTLEY

(KELSEY C. HARTLEY)

Copyright © 2019 (KELSEY C. HARTLEY)

All rights reserved

DISCLAIMER

All knowledge contained in this book is given for informational and educational purposes only. The author is not in any way accountable for any results or outcomes that emanate from using this material. Constructive attempts have been made to provide information that is both accurate and effective, but the author is not bound for the accuracy or use/misuse of this information.

Contents

DISCLAIMER iv

INTRODUCTION 1

CHAPTER ONE 5

THE CONCEPT OF HERBALISM... 5

WHAT ABOUT ESSENTIAL OILS?............................. 8

CHAPTER TWO 13

MAKING HERBAL MEDICINE FOR INTERNAL
USE 13

Food Herbs 16

METHODS OF MAKING INTERNAL HERBS 17

CHAPTER THREE 25

MAKING HERBAL MEDICINE FOR EXTERNAL
USE 25

CHAPTER FOUR **38**

COMBINING HERBS INTO A FORMULA 38

MOUTH/NOSE/EAR TREATMENT FORMULA . 42

GASTRO-INTESTINAL   TREATMENT
FORMULA... 43

LIVER/BILIARY TREATMENT FORMULA 45

RESPIRATORY TREATMENT FORMULA.............. 47

REPRODUCTIVE TREATMENT FORMULA 49

URINARY TRACT TREATMENT FORMULA 52

CARDIO-VASCULAR TREATMENT FORMULA .. 53

EXTERNAL HERB TREATMENT FORMULA....... 55

CENTRAL NERVOUS SYSTEM TREATMENT
FORMULA... 57

TREATMENT FORMULA FOR PLEASURE OR FUN
.... 59

CHAPTER FIVE **62**

IMPORTANT CONSIDERATIONS IN USING HERBAL
MEDICINE 62

CONCLUSION **68**

INTRODUCTION

They say *Health is Wealth*, and the way we manage our body is a significant determinant of the state of our health. Managing one's health deals with taking preventive measures against any form of sickness and diseases. It also involves knowing the right way to go when it comes to taking treatments when any ailments or diseases pop up. There have been different means of treating or preventing the occurrences of any form of illness in our body.

From time immemorial, the use of herbs to heal and prevent the different form of diseases and sicknesses was the order of the moment. They got these herbs from plants, tree barks, and seeds. The single-use or combination of any of these worked wonders. Whenever there was any form of health issue, the elders knew what kind of herbs to use to cure them. Each community had a known herbalist, whose profession was to identify different herbs and give directions on how to apply them for different uses. Herbal medicine was widely used in different parts of the world, most notably in Africa, China, Europe, India, Indonesia, and also the Northern and Southern America.

When a child is born, different types of herbs are used on the baby to keep him or her healthy. These herbs served as a preventive mechanism against any diseases that could pop up over time. During these periods, people truly believed in the effectiveness of these herbs. It never failed them in any way. The practice of herbal medicine flourished until the 17th century, when more scientific pharmacological inceptions became widely accepted.

The era of industrialization came, and inventions began to creep into the different sectors of people's life, and the health sector was not an exception. This led to the birthing of various pharmaceutical companies for the production of drugs. Patents were given to the pharmaceutical companies for the production of some medicines. People started buying into the latest trend, and the era of herbs began to fade out bit by bit. The scientific research that was backing the production of these pharmaceutical drugs were getting positive feedbacks because they were able to cure different diseases. Advancement came to these scientific methods in the 19th century, which led to the dismissal of the herbal process, referring to it as Quackery.

However, in recent times, the severity of the side effects of modern medicine led to the desire for a more self-reliance method and also a natural approach to human health. And this brought back an increased interest in herbal medicine. Also, the fact that the establishment of the Office of Alternative Medicine by the National Institute of Health in 1992, made herbal use a popular and viable method again. Also, in 1974, the World Health Organization encouraged developing the use traditional plant medicines as an alternative for the unmet desires from modern systems. Again, the use of herbal medicine has gained worldwide relevance.

The use of herbal medicine has been a notable way of life in China. They have been able to develop the production of their herbs, so that they come in capsules and teas. Although thirty percent of all modern drugs come from plants, we cannot compare the significance of these herbal drugs in their natural state with those of 'modern' medications. We can't help but see the evidence of the consistent use of herbs in China has done to the average health of every inhabitant. They live a healthy life, and they enjoy longevity. How else do you think that's possible? A herbal way of life, obviously.

The use of herbs have been studied in different disciplines, and this has made its advancement a possibility. Now, you could find different innovations coming with the study of herbs. You can enjoy herbs in the form of teas, powdered herbs, and essential oils. We are going to look deeper into all these throughout this book. All you need to do is relax and stay glued to this book, while I take you through the journey of knowing the importance and applications of different herbs and essential oils for a better quality life. I assure you that it's going to be such an amazing and enlightening experience going through this book. Have a great time reading!

CHAPTER ONE

THE CONCEPT OF HERBALISM

The use of herbs has in one way or the other spurred the need to do a more in depth study of it. And different professionals are taking time to study the significance of herbs in our immediate environment. You would agree that there is a need to know more about herbs, how it works, the good and bad sides of it, and how to develop these herbs in the best way possible. The quest to do all these gave way to the concept of *herbalism*.

Herbalism (also known as herbal medicine) is the study of medicinal plants in terms of how it is used and the understanding of their biological structure. Herbalism also refers to the folk and traditional therapeutic practice that is based on the use of plants and extracts from plants. Herbalism can also be referred to as *phytotherapy*. The use of herbs for the treatment of diseases is known to be widely used among non-industrialized societies. Some traditions in line with these societies give high regard to the practice of herbal medicine in the western world, at the end of the 20th century. In recent times, many of the pharmaceuticals available to Western physicians have a long history of the use of herbal remedies with the inclusion of aspirin, opium, digitalis, and quinine. This is as a result of the herbal contents found in those drugs.

All plants around us produce chemical compounds as a regular part of their metabolic activities, which can be grouped into two categories. The first is primary metabolites, which includes sugars and fats in all the plants. The second is secondary metabolites, which are found in a smaller variety of plants. There are variations in the autologous functions of secondary metabolites. Some of the features are: they serve as toxins that deter predation, or to attract insects for pollination. They also have therapeutic tasks in humans, in which they can be refined to produce drugs. Examples include quinine from the cinchona, inulin from the roots of dahlias, digoxin from the foxglove, morphine and codeine from the poppy. This is to show us that most of these modern drugs get their roots from these plants. Although, the need for a more natural approach to therapy brings herbalism as an effective alternative medicine. And this has resulted in increased demand, other than solely depending on the pharmaceutical drugs used in modern medicine that is synthetic.

The use of herbal medicine is common among patient with chronic diseases such as cancer, diabetes, asthma, and end-stage kidney disease. The different factors that have an association with the prevalence of herbal remedies include age, gender, ethnicity, education, and social status. The prescription drugs are usually sold alongside essential oils, herbal extracts, or herbal teas. Herbal remedies are seen by some to be the preferred form of treatment, other than pure medical compounds that have been industrially produced.

The practitioners of herbal medicine are known as herbalists. For them to get the level of an herbalist, they must learn the many skills including the wild crafting or cultivation of herbs, diagnosis, and treatment of conditions or dispensing herbal medication, and preparations of herbal medicines. The education of herbalists differs considerably in different parts of the world. For some locations, people generally rely upon an apprenticeship to becoming an herbalist in place of formal schooling. In some areas like the United Kingdom, the training of herbalists is done by state-funded universities offering a

Bachelor of Science degrees in herbal medicine. I believe that is a much more formal one.

Herbalists are known for their abilities to use extracts from parts of plants, such as the roots or leaves, believing that plants are subject to environmental pressures. And therefore develop resistance to threats such as radiation, reactive oxygen species, and microbial attack to survive. In the long run providing defensive phytochemicals of use in herbalism, which turns out to be a sustainable means of therapy for diseases.

WHAT ABOUT ESSENTIAL OILS?

There's no way we are going to talk about herbalism without looking into essential oils because they are birthed from the exploration of herbs for therapeutic purposes. Essential oils are concentrated hydrophobic liquid that contains volatile chemical compounds, which is gotten from plants. Essential oils can also be referred to as volatile oils, aetherolea oils or ethereal oils. Essential oils are derived from plant extracts.

Essential oils are called 'essential' because it contains the essence of the plant's fragrance – the fragrance of the plant from where it originated. The fact that it is called 'essential' does not mean it is indispensable. In contrast to fatty oils, essential oils naturally evaporate totally without leaving a stain or residue.

The mode of extraction of essential oils is generally by distillation, which is often done by using steam. Other processes involved include expression, full oil extraction, solvent extraction, *sfumatura*, wax embedding, cold pressing, and resin tapping. They are used in perfumes, soaps cosmetics, and other products. They are also used for flavoring food and drink, for adding fragrances to incense, and for household cleaning products.

Essential oils are commonly used for aromatherapy, which is a form of alternative medicine with healing effects that are ascribed to aromatic compounds. Aromatherapy is typically used to induce relaxation. Improper use of essential oils may be harmful to those using it – resulting in allergic reactions and skin irritation. Children may be particularly susceptible to the toxic effects of the improper use of essential oils.

Essential oils are usually lipophilic (*oil-loving*) compounds that cannot be mixed with water by default. They can be diluted in solvents like polyethylene glycol and pure ethanol. The most common way to safely dilute essential oils for topical use is in a carrier oil. This can be any vegetable oil freely available, and the most prevalent for skincare like coconut, olive, wheat germ, and avocado.

Some of the examples of essential oils include the following:

➢ **Balsam of Peru**

Balsam of Peru is an essential oil that is derived from the *Myroxylon*. It is used for flavoring in food and drink, for fragrance in perfumes and toiletries, and it has its healing properties in medicine and pharmaceutical items.

➢ **Eucalyptus Oil**

Most eucalyptus oil that we have in the market is produced from the leaves of *Eucalyptus globulus*. The steam-distilled eucalyptus oil is used throughout Asia, South America, Latin America, and Africa, as a primary cleaning/disinfecting agent added to soaped mop and countertop cleaning solutions. It also has insect and some degree of vermin control properties. However, there are hundreds of species of eucalyptus, and possibly some dozens are used to various extents as sources of essential oils. The products of different species do not only differ significantly in characteristics and effects, but also the outcomes of the same tree can vary utterly.

➤ Garlic Oil

Garlic oil is an essential oil that is derived from garlic as its source. It is a volatile oil prepared using steam distillation, which can also be manufactured by distillation. Garlic oil functions well in cooking as a seasoning, it serves as a nutritional supplement, and also can be used as an insecticide.

➤ Lavender Oil

Lavender oil has, for a long time, been used in the production of perfume. Lavender oil has the tendencies of being estrogenic and antiandrogenic. Thereby triggering problems for preadolescent boys and pregnant women precisely. The lavender essential oil can also be used as an insect repellent.

➤ Rose Oil

Rose oil is produced from the petals of *Rosa damascena* and *Rosa centifolia*. It is steam-distilled rose oil known as "rose otto," while the solvent extracted product is referred to as "rose absolute."

Some essential oils meet the requirements of *Generally Recognized as Safe (GRAS)*. Also, flavoring agents for use in foods, beverages, and confectioneries according to strict Good Manufacturing Practice (GMP) and flavorist standards. Some oils can be toxic to some domestic animals, with cats in particular. The internal use of essential oils can pose hazards to pregnant women. Some can be abortifacients in dose 0.5–10 mL, and thus should not be used during pregnancy.

CHAPTER TWO

MAKING HERBAL MEDICINE FOR INTERNAL USE

One thing to know is how to produce herbs; another thing is to understand the application of these herbs. The application of herbs is essential for anyone who wants to you use herbs for the cure of any ailment. You can't afford to drink herbs that are to be applied to your skin, doing that can be more hazardous than you can imagine. There are essential oils that you are meant to take into your system. And some are meant for the outer part of your body. You need to know how to distinguish them. This is the more reason why I'm here, to tell you all you need to know about different herbs that have internal importance, and how to go about it.

The internal use of herbs involve the types of herbs that will require you to ingest it. Some of the herbs are in the form of teas, powder, syrups, herbal juices, and essential oils. Also, some of these herbs, which are meant for our internal use, comes in the form of seasoning applied to the foods that we eat. These herbs enhance the taste and flavor of our foods. The health significance of the internal use of these herbs is multidimensional. Some serve as preventive measures against illnesses while some give the cure to the ailments like cancer, diabetes, cardiovascular diseases and other forms of terminal ailments. Here, we are going to talk about the making of some of these internal use herbs for our well-being.

How we make herbs have a way of affecting the way the herbs expresses itself. This is based on the actual constituents and the matter that is extracted, as well as the interactions that take place during the process of preparation. There overall connotation and the study of the plant, and its personality will make the processed herbs come through stronger. This is dependent on the way of preparation of the herbs, the person giving the medicine, and the recipient of the herbs.

Added to the healing process are other factors; the purposes of those making and administering the herbal medicine, and how the herbs that they put into the process will affect the outcome. The study of the individual that will be ingesting the herbal solution is of great importance. In any healing process, there is an interaction between the person seeking healing, the person holding the healing space and the medicine itself.

We are all aware of the fact that we bring forward different aspects of our personality when interacting with different people or groups of people and in various instances. The same applies to plants. Though, there may be broad similarities in the therapeutic effects of Lavender from individual plants of the species on most humans, there will also be variations and distinctions.

Part of the skills of working with the plants is to listen to the person who is seeking medicine, the time that you have and the situation you are working with – there are no absolutes.

We go deeper into our relationship with and our knowledge of the plants when we incorporate information such as the constituents, the properties, the general uses of these plants. We also sit with them to deepen our relationship with them, and we continue to do this as we do with dear friends, with people in our community. So, the plants are our allies and our teachers. We need to get to know them on every level and to ask them how we can work with them.

Food Herbs

One of the simplest and oldest ways of using herbs is to eat them as food. Hippocrates said, let your food be your medicine and your medicine be your food; well, we can do this with herbs. Dieting on herbs is the most excellent form of preventative medicine. It's a way of connecting properly with our environment and making ourselves more aligned with nature. Herbs are full of all sorts of nutrients which are anti-oxidant, anti-inflammatory, immune system and tissue building, cleansing and tonic to the blood, clearing for the liver and much more. Studies are emerging showing that including foraged foods and reasonable quantities of herbs and spices in the diet are preventative and curative for most of the ailments of Western culture such as diabetes, high blood pressure, high cholesterol, chronic inflammatory disease in general.

Kids love the frisson of preparing food from 'weeds' and wild plants. Many of our most valuable native and naturalized plants can be included in our diet effortlessly. They are much easier to grow, they are fresher, in season, totally local and are flavorsome.

METHODS OF MAKING INTERNAL HERBS

Like I have discussed earlier in this section, the ways and manner in which we prepare herbs differ based on the type and nature of the herbs. There are different methods of making internal herbs for different kinds of herbs. I have brought together some essentials of these herbs and the peculiarity of how they are prepared below:

➢ **Teas**

Teas, tisanes or infusions are probably the next oldest way of using herbs, and one of the easiest ways of using them. They are generally prepared from leaves, flowers, aerial parts, and some seeds. Either fresh or dried; they can also be prepared from powders of harder plant parts such as roots, barks, and seeds. Teas will mainly extract the water-soluble components of the plant. If you are using an aromatic plant (one containing essential oil) use a teapot, or place a saucer over the cup while infusing. Always use freshly boiled water. Some plants are used as a substitute for tea, and up to 5 cups can be safely consumed in a day.

However, I would recommend that if being used in this way, a maximum number per day would be 3-4 for any single herb. Use a variety of herbs from day to day or during the day other than just one (unless you are dieting with a particular plant to get to know it better). Some herbs are much stronger in their action and are not suited for food use, these should be taken less often in the day.

The standard way to prepare a tea is to use one teaspoon of dried herb or two teaspoons of fresh herbs (or a mixture of herbs) for one cup; pour on boiling water and allow the herbs to infuse for 5-10 minutes. If you are preparing a pot use 20g of dried herb or 30g of fresh herbs to 500 ml of water. Infusions can be stored in a covered container in the fridge for up to 24 hours. They may also be made in a thermos flask and stored in this for 24 hours.

Do not add milk as this may bind some of the active constituents. Try to take without sweetening since the taste of the herbs has healing qualities and informs the gut-brain and vagus nerve of the plant's medicine, but if necessary add a small amount of honey or apple juice concentrate.

Cold infusions are used for herbs containing large amounts of mucilage, e.g., Althea officinalis Marshmallow, linseed, and psyllium. Aromatic herbs; those containing significant amounts of essential oil are sometimes also extracted by cold infusion. Soaking in cold water for 12 hours, this can be good if a cooling effect is being sought. An example is the making of cold Tilia linden blossom infusion to calm hot flushes.

Teas can be prepared from a single species, or you can experiment with blending herbs in a tea. There are some examples in the profiles, but this can be an incredibly creative process and encourages us to work with taste, smell, and the appearance of the tea.

➢ Herbal Juices

Herbal Juices can be purchased or prepared with a suitable juicer at home. You need to use a wheatgrass juicer, rather than the juicers sold for making fruit and vegetable juices. They need to be prepared fresh or frozen if stored for more than 24 hours. This can be done in ice cube trays. The standard dose for juices is 5-10 ml 2-3 times per day.

➢ Powders

Powders are an alternative to the liquid forms for internal use and can also be used in external preparations. Once an herb is powdered, it is more susceptible to oxidation because it has larger surface area which is exposed to the air. This means that powders need to be kept in airtight containers and be used before they lose their potency. Powders are a great way to use herbs for adding into food; they can be sprinkled on soups or other foods, added to smoothies, or used to prepare infusions. They can also be used to pack capsules. Capsule fillers are available from various sources online. Capsules suitable for vegans and vegetarians and are available from several suppliers. The standard dose is 2-3 capsules twice a day – this dose contains about 250 mg of the herb. The equivalent amount of powdered herb could also be sprinkled on food.

➢ Glycerites

Vegetable Glycerin is produced by the hydrolysis of vegetable fats, most commonly palm or coconut oil. It is better to use vegetable glycerin rather than animal glycerin or glycerin that has been chemically synthesized. Or those produced from other less desirable sources such as the petrochemical industry.

Glycerine is both a solvent and a preservative in the same way as alcohol, although it is not a quite as useful solvent, like alcohol. It sits somewhere between alcohol and water as a solvent and likewise in its efficiency as a preservative. Another way of looking at this is to say glycerine can extract a broader range of constituents but at lower levels. It does, however, have a wide range of applications in herbal medicine and is the perfect choice when looking to manufacture alcohol-free preparations.

A glycerite is a preparation that uses glycerin to extract the constituents from a herb in a similar fashion as to how one would use alcohol when making a tincture. Glycerites can be produced from both fresh and dry herbs using different ratios for extraction purposes.

Dry Herb Glycerite: Specification: 1:5 at 60% 1kg herb to 5 liters of liquid, 60% of which is glycerin and 40% water

Fresh Herb Glycerite: Specification 1:2 at 70% 1kg herb to 2 liters of liquid, 70% of which is glycerin and 30% water

A higher percentage of glycerin is used with fresh herbs due to the higher water content of the herbs.

Method

- Weigh herbs and place in a glass jar or pail, label with specification and contents.

- Measure glycerin and add to the jar

- Measure water and add to the jar

- Shake well

- Allow macerating for 28 days shaking each day to distribute the liquid

- Press the herb and glycerin mixture into another jar, discarding the marc

- After a couple of days decant the glycerite into a dark bottle and label.

- Store in a cool place out of direct sunlight

Warm Glycerite Method: Dry Herb Specification: 1:5 Fresh Herb Specification 1:2 using neat vegetable glycerin

Method

- Place your herbs in a clean glass jar

- Cover with glycerin

- Cover with lid

- Place a folded dishcloth in the bottom of a saucepan or crockpot

- Place your jar on top of the cloth

- Fill your saucepan or crockpot full of water – cover as much of your jar as possible

- Cook on low heat for three days refilling water as it evaporates

- Shake 2-3 times a day

- Strain herbs through a cheesecloth or muslin and dispose of them in the compost heap

- Store the liquid in a glass jar, label, and keep in a cool, dark place

- A glycerite made using this method will typically last about one year when stored properly.

The fresh glycerite is considered to be a more efficient product than a dry glycerite. The extraction process releases more constituents and has better preservative qualities. This is due to the increased "toughness" of the cellular wall in a dry herb which can compromise extraction and preservation. However, both fresh and dry glycerites have their applications, and there is empirical evidence to support both methods of extraction. The hot process of manufacturing glycerites produces a product more akin to an herbal syrup, concentrated, effective, and quicker to make than the cold techniques.

A glycerite should contain between 55-70% glycerin to prevent deterioration and potential mold growth during storage. When manufacturing a fresh herb glycerite, a standard of 70% will ensure the water content of the final product is not too high and thus preventing a risk of breakdown.

These are some of the herbs for internal use and the making of them. Whenever we are making herbs, we need to put in cognizance to the peculiarities of these herbs. The different ways that they are produced should be considered. Also, the way they are administered and the importance each of these herbs has on our health. Knowing this will enable us to be able to know what type of herbs to use to cure a particular form of ailment at a specific point in time.

CHAPTER THREE

MAKING HERBAL MEDICINE FOR EXTERNAL USE

L ike we discussed in the previous section, it is a thing to know the function of different herbs and it is another to understand how to produce the herbs. But it is yet another thing to understand the best application of these herbs that have been produced. Herbs have been a blessing to us from time immemorial. In different parts of the world, there are various forms of herbs peculiar to the different locations of those different parts of the world. For example, Ginseng is one of the herbs that is predominantly traced to China. These herbs have the unique properties that make them stand out and used for which it was designed.

On the use of herbs, there is internal use, and there is external use. Internal use is the one we take in (whether by drinking or eating), in the form of herbal juice, powder, teas, food herbs (vegetables), syrups, and essential oils. The external use being the subject of discussion here are the ones that involve you apply on the outer parts of your body. You cannot afford to make a costly mistake of using external use herbs for internal purposes as this can bring harmful adverse effects to your body. The more reason why it is crucial for us understanding the peculiarity of each herb and how they are used. External herbs usually come out stronger than the internal herbs based on the process used in making these herbs, and also the nature of these herbs.

External herbs come in the form of soaps, creams, balms, powders, liquefied herbs, and essential oils. We know for a fact that the soaps are meant to be used while we take our baths. The liquefied herbs are also used for different forms of herbal baths. And the creams are intended to be rubbed on our skin. The balms and essential oils are the ones usually applied to some specific parts of the skin. This is to show that some of these external herbs are used for a different therapeutic purpose. And these involve curing skin diseases such as psoriasis, acne, skin rashes, pimples, and skin poxes. They also have relieving effects on the body from any form of bone pains or muscle aches or any skin injury. Some are applied for clearer visual effects. How they are made is also of importance. We need to be enlightened on the ways and manners involved in producing these herbs. And in this chapter, we are going to look into the different methods involved. And styles of making some of these herbs for external therapeutic purposes.

Baths

Bathing with herbs has been a lifelong tradition. In Ireland, there are still several places that offer seaweed baths for health. Herbal baths can be used for many purposes. Footbaths are good for detoxifying the system and stimulating the circulation. Hand baths can be valuable for arthritic hands. Full body baths can be great for delivering a good dose of herbs transdermally (through the skin). Our skin is permeable to many of the plants' constituents, and they get straight into the general circulation. Sitz baths are used to treat the bowel, kidneys, reproductive organs, and congestion in the abdomen and pelvis and problems with the hips. For a sitz bath one needs two containers that are large enough to sit in. One contains hot water with the herbs or oils added, the other contains cold water. One sits first in hot water and herbs with the feet in the cold water so that the circulation and the medicine are drawn into the lower trunk for about 10 minutes.

Then one sits in the cold water with the feet in hot water for 10 minutes to bring the circulation to the extremities. This can be repeated several times. Baths can be prepared with infusions, decoctions or essential oils and salt or Epsom salts may also be used.

➢ Poultices

Poultices are made with a mixture of fresh, dried or powdered herbs, simmered or steeped in the minimum quantity of water for two minutes and applied externally. Marshmallow root powder, green clay, or linseed can be added to give a better texture and for their drawing qualities, especially for infected wounds, ulcers or boils. Poultices are also used for nerve and muscle pain, sprains, and broken bones. In these cases, a small pinch of ginger or a couple of drops of ginger oil may be added to 'potentize' the action. Poultices may also be used for mastitis or engorged breasts- either cold cabbage leaves or warm calendula. Try to ensure that only sufficient water is present when simmering or soaking in hot water to form a firm texture without having to squeeze off any liquid. Apply some oil to the area being treated to prevent the poultice sticking, and the herbs are applied as hot as possible, taking care not to scald the skin. The herbs are laid on lint and covered with gauze, then the poultice is applied, gauze side to the skin and bandaged in place. It may be left for between 30 minutes and 24 hours, depending on what is being treated.

➢ Aromatic Waters

Aromatic waters are also known as hydrosols, hydrolats, distillates, floral waters or flower waters. They are the water phase of steam distillation, saturated with water-soluble volatile components such as alcohols and acids. These have their therapeutic properties and are widely used in continental Europe. Aromatic waters can be prepared from herbs that do not contain any essential oil too. In France and other countries on the continent, many rural households will have a small still for making this sort of medicine to use at home. Hydrosols are used internally at a similar standard to tinctures; they can also be used externally as skin washes, and as ingredients in creams or compresses. They are also used in cooking. N.B. Mixing distilled water and essential oils does not produce the same product. For home use, aromatic waters can be prepared using a pressure cooker or a preserving pan.

➢ Macerated or Infused oils

Macerated or infused oils are made by soaking the herb in cold-pressed unrefined vegetable oil (almond, olive, sunflower are commonly used) for several weeks. The purpose is to obtain a cold infusion or by gently heating to about 60°C. Cover a water bath for about three hours for a hot infusion. Once the maceration process is complete, the oil is put through a press to complete the extraction and remove the spent herb. This process extracts the fat-soluble components of the herbs for use in massage oils, lotions, creams, and ointments. If a stronger preparation is required, then the process is sometimes repeated with a fresh batch of the herb. They will keep for up to a year if stored in a cool, dry place.

Hot method

250g dried or 500g fresh herb

750ml cold-pressed virgin and preferably organic vegetable oil (olive oil is the most stable for heating.

- Mix the chopped herbs and oil in a pyrex bowl and place over a pan of boiling water. Cover and simmer gently for 2-3 hours.

- Remove from the heat and allow to cool. Then pour into a winepress as described for the vinegar, or through a muslin bag.

- Collect the strained oil in a sterile jug and pour into sterilized bottles — label with date and contents.

- Store in a cool dark place for up to 1 year.

Cold method

1. Loosely pack a sterile jar with fresh or dried herb. Herbs with a high water content such as calendula, chickweed, basil or comfrey are best prepared with dried herb, or by the hot method to prevent them from going rancid. St. John's Wort is best made by the cold process.

2. Place the jar on a sunny windowsill or in the hot press and leave for 2-6 weeks.

3. Strain as described for vinegar.

4. Label and stored as described above.

Infused oils may be used for culinary purposed, as massage oils or as the base to prepare ointments and creams.

➢ Ointments/salves/balms

Ointments/salves/balms are oil-based mixtures that help to protect the skin and only contain oily ingredients. They can be thickened with any wax, including paraffin wax, but beeswax is preferable as it has its therapeutic proprieties. Use unbleached beeswax. If beeswax is not available use cocoa butter or another plant wax/or fat. Previously duck or goose fat and pig lard have been used and would be deemed to have their therapeutic benefits. Ointments stay on the skin for a long time, so they are useful for forming barriers to protect the skin. They are also healing and soothing. They are good for nappy rash, and for protecting the lips. They are also useful for dry areas such as knees, heels, feet, and elbows.

They also keep heat and water in, good for rheumatic aches, dehydrated skin and conditions made worse by cold weather. Do not use them if the skin is hot, inflamed, or weepy.

300 ml infused oil or base oil

25 g beeswax; shredded or in beads.

Warm the ingredients together in a bain-marie just to the point where the waxes melt. Add essential oils if desired and pour into clean jars. Label and leave to set in the fridge.

➢ Plasters

Plasters are made by spreading the ointment onto the clean bandage. Cover the dressing with a layer of cling film or oilcloth and roll up to store. Place in an airtight container in the fridge, or a cool, dry place. Label with the ingredients and date. They are a convenient way of applying ointment to aching joints etc. All these preparations should be used within 9-12 months.

➢ Creams

Creams are lighter than ointments, as they contain water and oil in an emulsion. Creams are more cooling than ointments and are absorbed more quickly. They are more suitable for hot, inflamed and weepy skin conditions. They are also useful for applying to warm areas of the body, such as the groin. The ones described below are water in oil emulsions, which are good for moisturizing. Oil in water emulsions is more difficult to make at home. A basic cream can be made with:

50 ml of oil

15 g beeswax

50 ml water/ infusion/decoction/ floral water/ tincture

Galen's Cold cream

40 g almond oil

10 g beeswax

40 g rose water

10 drops essential oil

Cocoa buttercream

50 g calendula oil

35 g cocoa butter

10 g beeswax

45 g floral water

25 drops essential oil

Coconut oil cream

50 g virgin coconut oil

20 g almond oil

25 g floral water/infusion

20 drops essential oil

Cream method:

Make sure ingredients are weighed accurately in a clean scales. Otherwise, the consistency will be affected. If beeswax is being used, then shred finely before considering or use beads. Put oily and fatty ingredients into a stainless steel or pyrex bowl (oils, beeswax, cocoa butter, etc.) Put wet ingredients – floral waters, spring water, decoction, infusion or tincture into a separate stainless steel or pyrex bowl and stand both jars in a shallow pan of water or bain-marie over a gentle heat. Liquid lecithin can be added to the oily ingredients to help emulsification, and borax can be added to the wet ingredients for the same effect. Stir the bowl with the fatty ingredients to facilitate melting, remove both jars from the heat. The best way to form an emulsion is to use an electric egg beater on its' lowest speed. Alternatively, use an egg whisk or a balloon whisk. Add the water slowly (a few drops at a time, increasing to a small stream), until it is all incorporated – like making mayonnaise. When all the water has been added stop beating at once, too much beating can make the cream separate. If adding essential oils, stir in carefully. The cream can then be put into jars and left in the fridge until set. Make sure to label jars with ingredients and date. The cream can also be divided into several jars and different essential oils added to the individual jars.

Formulae can be multiplied up to make larger batches of cream. Once the technique has been mastered, you can also play around with the proportions to make lighter or firmer creams – enjoy.

To increase the shelf life part of the oily ingredients can be substituted with wheat germ oil, or with vitamin E oil. The base oil can also be varied to give a different quality of the cream. Essential oils that are particularly good for preserving the creams are lavender, tea tree or benzoin. None of these are as effective as the preservatives that are used in commercial creams, but they will give a longer shelf life. Storing in the fridge will also lengthen shelf life. Also, rather than dipping fingers into the jars use a spatula or spoon to dispense the cream.

Before making any of these preparations, you need to prepare your equipment and ensure that it is spotlessly clean. Use stainless steel, or glass containers, bowls, and pans. Use stainless steel implements, for stirring, mixing, chopping ingredients, and so on.

Avoid using any dirty jars, or implements, tie back long hair, and keep fingers out of all mixtures to prevent contamination. Any preparations that show signs of contamination (mold growing or smelling 'off') should be discarded immediately. Occasionally, water will 'bleed' out of the cream. This does not mean that they have gone off, but that some separation has occurred. They are still ok to use.

CHAPTER FOUR

COMBINING HERBS INTO A FORMULA

I n the introductory part of this book, I talked about the concept of herbalism in the different countries of the world, and I emphasized the Chinese culture of herbal medicine. You might be wondering why I did that, but do you know that the Chinese have a reputation for living long and leaving healthy? How do you think that is possible except for their herbal lifestyle? When you talk about combining herbs into different herbal formulas, then you are going to talk about the usual Chinese method of herbal combination taking the front row, which I believe that other continents of the world should imbibe for a healthy living.

Combining herbs into a formula is a process that involves bringing different herbs together in a definite proportion to bring a lasting cure to various forms of ailments. The thing about these herbs is that they have chemical properties that come in similar forms, and combining them brings about effective results. The modern western pharmacology tends to focus on finding the single-molecule that cures a disease. In contrast, Chinese medicine often utilizes herbal formulas that blend many agents to address underlying imbalances that may cause illness while aiding in symptom relief – a 'shotgun' approach that has been practiced in Asia for thousands of years. Medical practitioners all over the world have begun to incorporate more Chinese formulas into their practices to treat common, everyday conditions. Whereas raw herbs were once sent home with the patient and made into teas, today there are a variety of forms available over the counter, in practitioners' offices and in health food stores.

The combination of herbal formulas deals with the different methods used in bringing these herbs together to form a practical whole for therapeutic purposes. Speaking of which ***Decoction*** is a significant order, when it comes to the process of combining herbs into a formula. We can give speculations on the origins of decoctions. But it is easy enough to imagine that if you wanted to try to consume a food or medicinal herbal material that was tough, there was little choice but to cook it up in the water and drink the resulting liquid. And, possibly, eat the softened material that had been boiled for a long time. Converting the herb (or animal or mineral) to a powder was not an option for most individuals. That would require first taking the time to dry the substance thoroughly and then make an effort to reduce it to powder by some simple means (such as was used to make flour from grains; though grains are a lot easier to powder than many other natural materials). Perhaps at an Imperial herbal pharmacy, one would have enough impetus and enough labor to produce some powders and store them up for when they need to be used. Making powder is not a spur of the moment option (though administering the already produced powders is), processing a decoction could be done relatively quickly and easily.

Decoctions were the dominant form of therapy in the **Shang Han Lun**, though other forms were mentioned, including powders and pills. This seems appropriate given the situation and the methodology in the text. The situation was a rapidly progressing disease that could easily cause death if not adequately treated. And the method was to adjust the formulation, often by changing only an herb or two, as the symptoms changed. Often, time was of the essence, and one might not wish to use a premade formula. Further, some of the essential prescriptions were intended to induce perspiration, and the hot liquid form helped bring about that result.

In the late 1970s and throughout the 1980s, decoctions were used by U.S. practitioners when Chinese herbal training was first available. But reliance on this method has declined somewhat for several reasons, including the widespread availability of other forms deemed more convenient by practitioners and patients. Most often, herb decoctions are prescribed by Chinese immigrants who have prior training and experience in using this form and who are comfortable with designing herb formulas for each patient.

Chinese medicine has become much more mainstream in its use and indications. Over-the-counter products are now used based on their modern-day disease indications and are used in their traditional applications for treating imbalances in organ channels. While modern medicine has tried to extract the most active components of herbs in an attempt to enhance their effects, Chinese herbal formulas continue to combine whole herbs. It is common to see herbs and minerals such as licorice, ginger, a simple sugar, rice, and salt added to help make the other components in a formula work better.

Having discussed Chinese medicine and decoctions, let us further look into the different formulas that are used in tackling the various forms of ailments. And these formulas are not limited to the Chinese alone; it is widespread. The processes and importance are also discussed in the outline below:

MOUTH/NOSE/EAR TREATMENT FORMULA

A. LIP and SKIN BUTTER

Almond Oil .... 20 ounces

Anhydrose Lanolin .... 1/2 pound

Glycerin .... 8 ounces

Beeswax .... 3 $^{3/4}$ ounces

5-10 drops of Essential Oil

Over low heat, dissolve the lanolin in the almond oil, add the glycerin and stir until all three are dispersed. Add the finely-chopped beeswax, stirring until just melted, add the essential oil, and pour the salve into containers. Stir the pot frequently and pour as quickly as possible. If you take too long, the lanolin and glycerin may begin to separate.

B. TOOTH POWDER

Orris Root Powder............. 4 ounces

Arrowroot ....4 ounces

Myrrh Gum.......................... 2 ounces

Licorice Root........................ 1.5 ounces

White Oak Bark .... 1.5 ounces

Golden Seal Root ....1 ounce

Bistort Root.......................... 1 ounce

Peppermint Oil .... 1/2 teaspoon

Mix powdered herbs thoroughly with Peppermint Oil.

GASTRO-INTESTINAL TREATMENT FORMULA

A. STOMACH TEA

Star Anise............................. 3 parts

Ginger Root.......................... 2 parts

Papaya Leaf.......................... 2 parts

Fennel Seed .... 2 parts

Camomile ....2 parts

Comfrey Leaf....................... 2 parts

Peppermint (or Poleo)........ 2 parts

Angelica or Calamus .... 1 part

As a simple infusion, as needed for dyspepsia or mild gastritis.

B. LAXATIVE TEA

Psyllium Seed...................... 3 parts

Licorice Root ....…... 3 parts

Rhubarb Root.................... 2 parts

Senna Pods (crushed) ...... 2 parts

Angelica Root .... 2 parts

Drink as a simple infusion in the evening.

C. COLON TONIC (Modified Thomsonian)

Cascara Sagrada .... 2 parts

Oregon Grape .... 2 parts

Cayenne .... 1 part

Ginger Root........................... 1 part

Lobelia.................................... 1 part

Rhubarb Root........................ 1 part.

Stimulates peristalsis for chronic constipation of long duration. 2 "00" caps with water, morning and evening. When feces soften up go to 1 capsule twice a day.

D. BITTER TONIC

Gentian Root 2 parts

Quassia Wood......................2 parts

(Or Castela)........................ (2 parts)

Angelica Root/Seed............2 parts

Cardamon Seed................... 1/2 part

Bayberry Bark...................... 1/2 part

Tincture 1:4, 50% alcohol. Best for chronic conditions, such as recovering anorectics, achlorhydria, chemotherapy queasiness. Take 5-15 drops 10-15 minutes before a meal.

LIVER/BILIARY TREATMENT FORMULA

A. LIVER TONIC

Barberry or Oregon Grape …….. 2 parts

Milk Thistle Seed............................. 2 parts

Chaparral (Larrea)........................... 1 part

Toadflax (Linaria)........................... 1 part

Echinacea.. 1 part

Burdock Root or Seed .... 1 part

Yellow Dock.................................... 1 part

Leptandra or Blue Flag Root ...... 1 part

An old-fashioned "shotgun" formula. Grind well and encapsulate. Echinacea is the only one of these herbs that deteriorates in a powdered form, so the best compromise would be to keep it as a rather coarse grind, the rest as fine a powder as desired. Useful for passive liver "heaviness," with periodic light stools and frontal headaches brought on by overeating or eating rich foods when tired. Look for greasy hair, acne on the cheeks (both kinds of cheeks) and acne around the mouth. It should be tried for those that regularly work with solvents or that drink regularly, whether in moderation or excess. In general, for those that regularly eat before going to bet and are slow in waking, grouchy and sluggish in the morning. They also have to cut back on the snacks.

DOSE: Pronounced liver dysfunction, but with or without pathology: 2 caps, 3 times a day. No overt symptoms, but having many of the risks mentioned: 1 cap, 3times a day.

B. ALTERATIVE TEA

Sassafrass Bark.................... 2 parts

Sarsaparilla Root................. 2 parts

Burdock Root....................... 1 part

Echinacea Root.................... 1 part

A simple, drinkable tea for low-level chronic liver, metabolic, and immunosuppressed states. Take a couple of cups a day, made from a rounded teaspoon in 8 ounces of water, brought to a boil and removed from the heat and allowed to cool.

RESPIRATORY TREATMENT FORMULA

A. DECONGESTANT TEA

Ma Huang .... 3 parts

Mormon Tea .... 3 parts

Yerba Santa....................................... 3 parts

Coltsfoot Leaves.............................. 3 parts

Cubeb Berries................................... 2 parts

Drink frequently as an infusion. If you find it interferes with sleep or makes you jittery, lessen or delete the Ma Huang.

B. WHITE PINE COMPOUND COUGH SYRUP

White Pine Bark (or Balsam Root) .... 3 ounces.

Wild Cherry Bark .... 3 ounces.

Spikenard Root .... 1/2 ounce

Poplar Buds .... 1/2 ounce

Blood Root .... 1/4 ounce

Percolate with 50% alcohol until you have reached 16 ounces. Add 12 ounces of simple syrup.

OR add 8 ounces of honey and 4 ounces of glycerin.

C. TONSILITIS FORMULA

Red Root .... 4 parts

Myrrh .... 2 parts

Bayberry .... 2 parts

Make from the individual tinctures, add 5% glycerin. Take 1/2 teaspoon in 2 tablespoons of hot water, gargle well and swallow every 2 hours.

REPRODUCTIVE TREATMENT FORMULA

A. FEMALE BALANCER

Vitex agnus-castus Tinct.... ....3 parts

Black Cohosh Tinct............ ....2 parts

Dandelion FE....................... ....2 parts

Motherwort Tinct............... ....2 parts

Oregon Grape Root Tinct...............1 part

Mix with fluid extracts and tinctures. Use 30-60 drops (1 or 2 squirts) 2 or 3 times a day. This helps to regulate chronically short estrus cycles, with aggravated anabolic metabolism.

B. MENOPAUSE: EARLY FORMULA

Vitex agnus-castus Tinct .... 3 parts

Yellow Dock Tinct .... 2 parts

Sarsaparilla Tinct .... 2 parts

Peony Tinct .... 2 parts

Nuphar Tinct .... 1 part

American Ginseng Tinct .... 1 part

Mix using tinctures, since some are best fresh, some best dry. Use 30-60 drops (1 or 2 squirts) 2 or 3 times a day. For women in earlier stages of menopause when erratic cycles and flooding result from increasingly disorganized corpus luteal progesterone production.

C. MENOPAUSE: LATER FORMULA

Motherwort .... 3 parts

Devil's Club .... 3 parts

Black Cohosh .... 2 parts

Licorice .... 2 parts

Bugleweed .... 2 parts

Dong Quai .... 1 part

Blue Cohosh ....…..... 1 part

Mix from tinctures or make 1:5, 60% alcohol. Use 30-60 drops (1 or 2 squirts) 2 or 3 times a day. For women in the later stages of menopause when ovulation has nearly ceased. And the main symptoms arise not from erratic progesterone levels, but from the hypothalamus and pituitary attempts to increase diminished estrogen levels.

D. HAYDEN'S VIBURNUM COMPOUND

Black Haw (V. prunifolium) .... 1.5 ounces

Cramp Bark (V. opulus) .... 1.0 ounce

Trillium (dried) .... 1.0 ounce

(OR Cotton Root Bark .... (1.0 ounce)

Dioscorea (Wild Yam) .... 1/2 ounce

Skullcap (recently dried) .... 1/4 ounce

Cloves ….. 1.0 ounce

Cinnamon Bark .... 3/4 ounce

Orange Peel .... 1/2 ounce

Grind herbs together, moisten with a few tablespoons of alcohol and let sit, covered, overnight. Tincture with 50% alcohol menstruum to a 1:4 tincture (about 26 ounces). Add 6.5 ounces (by volume) of Simple Syrup to bring the final strength to 1:5. You MAY substitute equal parts of glycerin and honey for the syrup, but it tastes weird. Take 1-3 teaspoons in HOT water for Killer Cramps, particularly if it is a problem that only happens every few months, or occurs only the first night of menstruation. Regular monthly dysmenorrhea from organic causes, rarely responds very well to H.V.C. This formula is the Queen of Cramp Remedies.

URINARY TRACT TREATMENT FORMULA

A. URINARY TINCTURE

Buchu Leaves .... 3 parts

Juniper berries .... 2 parts

Yerba Mansa .... 2 parts

Pipsissewa .... 2 parts

Eryngium yuccafolium .... 1 part

Mix as tinctures or make 1:5, with 65% alcohol. Use 30-60 drops (1 or 2 squirts) in 8 ounces of water, 3-4 times a day. A general diuretic and antimicrobial for water retention and mild urinary tract infections.

B. ALKALIZING TEA

Nettle Leaf .... 1 part

Red Clover Tops .... 1 part

Alfalfa .... 1 part

Horsetail (optional) .... 1 part

Drink hot or cold tea freely. If under metabolic stress, you might even use the tea as your main liquid. Suitable for acid urine, uric acid kidney stones, post-op recovery, PMSl acidity and as part of an osteoporosis regimen.

CARDIO-VASCULAR TREATMENT FORMULA

A. GREASEBALL HYPERTENSION

Equisetum.... ....4 parts

Dandelion Root................................4 parts

Passion Flower................................3 parts

Crataegus..2 parts

Prickly Ash.......................................2 parts

Capsicum...1 part

Aristolochia serpentaria..... ....1 part

Tincture 1:4 with 50% alcohol, after setting two days moistened. 1/2 teaspoon two times a day, with a blood anti-viscosity agent, such as Red Root, Vitamin E or an Aspirin.

B. HYPOTENSION FORMULA (Kidney deficient)

Kola Nuts .... 4 parts

Gotu Kola .... 3 parts

Licorice Root .... 2 parts

Korean red Ginseng .... 2 parts

Lily-of-the-Valley Root .... 1 part

Tincture 1:4, 50% alcohol 1/2 teaspoon in the morning and midday.

C. TACHYCARDIA FORMULA

Lycopus .... 3 parts

Leonurus .... 3 parts

Passiflora .... 2 parts

Crataegus .... 2 parts

Tincture 50%, 1:4 30-60 drops, 4 times a day.

D. CIRCULATORY STIMULANT

Prickly Ash Bark .... 3 parts

Ginger .... 2 parts

Immortal Root .... 2 parts

Osha Root .... 2 parts

Capsicum.............................1 part

Tincture 60%, 1:4 20-40 drops, 4 times a day. Thirty drops before meals as a bitter tonic, 30 drops before retiring.

EXTERNAL HERB TREATMENT FORMULA

A. CHAC SALVE (Calendula, Hypericum, Arnica, Cajeput)

Calendula Flowers	2 ounces
Arnica Herb	2 ounces
Ethanol	2 ounces
Olive Oil	24 ounces
Hypericum Oil	6 ounces
Cajeput Oil	1/2 ounces
Beeswax	5 ounces

Make a 1:6 steeped oil with the Calendula and Arnica (as usual), add the Hypericum Oil (made from the fresh flowers), heat slowly, dissolve the beeswax, add the Cajeput (actually Tea Tree Oil, but much cheaper by the older name), and pour into tins. Can also be called OSFA Salve (One Size Fits All) or Rescue Grease or Limbaugh Leech.

B. MUSCLE BALM

Poplar Bud Oil (steeped)	2 ounces
Arnica Oil (steeped)	2 ounces

Hypericum Oil (steeped) .... 2 ounces

Oil of Wintergreen .... 30 drops

Olive Oil .... 6 ounces

A Topical oil, used as an analgesic, counterirritant, and anti-inflammatory. 30-60 drops rubbed into the area aids dispersal and resolution of exudates. It is too strong for true massage oil.

C. ECHINACEA SALVE

Echinacea Purpurea Flowers .... 5 ounces

Alcohol .... 3 ounces

Olive Oil .... 35 ounces

Beeswax .... 7 ounces

Grind and sift the Echinacea Flowers (roots will not work). Mix the alcohol with the flowers in a stainless steel bowl with a lid, cover and let stand for at least 2-3 hours. Blend the moist herb with olive oil in a hearty blender until the container gets warm. Filter through muslin, squeezing the marc as well as possible, and heat the oil slowly in the top of a double boiler. Chop and add the beeswax, continuing the low heat until the beeswax has melted. Pour into containers. Use freely for hemorrhoids, blisters, cold sores, stings, vaginitis, anal fissures, and any inflamed swellings.

CENTRAL NERVOUS SYSTEM TREATMENT FORMULA

A. RELAXING TEA

Camomile Flowers .... 3 parts

Catnip .... 3 parts

Passion Flower .... 3 parts

Spearmint .... 2 parts

Lemon Balm .... 2 parts

Hops .... 2 parts

Viscum album .... 1 part

Drink the simple infusion as needed, particularly in the evenings. If you know you will have trouble sleeping, start drinking it BEFORE you can't sleep.

B. NERVE TONIC

Valerian .... 4 parts

Verbena .... 4 parts

Skullcap .... 4 parts

Passion Flower .... 4 parts

European Mistletoe .... 2 parts

Damiana .... 2 parts

Siberian Ginseng .... 2 parts

Corydalis .... 1 part

Use 3-6 capsules as needed. Lower doses help anxieties, and larger doses act as an overt sedative. (Can be tinctured, 50% alcohol)

C. SPEED DETOX FORMULA

Bee Pollen .... 6 parts

Fu-Tze (Cured Aconite) ...... 4 parts

Mahonia .... 3 parts

Use 6-12 caps a day with 250 mg. of tyrosine a day and water-soluble vitamins such as B complex and C. Used to help someone get through the first week of amphetamine or cocaine withdrawal.

TREATMENT FORMULA FOR PLEASURE OR FUN

A. MESOMARBLES

Bee Pollen .... 8 parts

Guarana .... 2 parts

Korean "Red" Ginseng .... 1 part

Powder together and take pinches as food, or mix with a little honey and form balls.

B. GUARANA FUDGE (AKA Speed Fudge)

Mix: .... 5 cups brown sugar

.... 2 $^{1/2}$ cups of milk

.... Salt

Add later: .... 1 cube sweet butter

.... 6 ounces powdered Guarana Bean

.... Various nuts (if desired

Boil to the softball stage. Remove from heat for 10 minutes, add one sweet cube butter. Mix in 6 ounces of powdered Guarana Bean, and continuously stir until the glistening surface starts to look like frosting and stiffens. Add nuts (if desired), scrape onto a greased surface, cool until set, and cut.

WARNING: This stuff tastes GREAT, but speeds like a light. There are no self-redeeming qualities to this; instead, it's just happily perverse. You must be careful to take in moderation.

Dosage: start with a small square, and wait an hour before overlapping with another piece. Guarana is the Queen of caffeine plants (with some hypoxanthine thrown in). And it will generally produce gayety, restlessness, quick perception, and wakefulness while slowing the pulse and impairing the appetite. Eating it slows absorption and can extend its effects well past the 3-4 hours you might expect from a similar amount of coffee. The fudge tastes good; the impact of Guarana is fun. But if you overeat this stuff, you can get to a level of pure caffeine jitters that completely overrides the subtleties that, at a more reasonable amount, make Guarana so lovely.

We can see from all these formulas that they are special in their combinations, and the therapeutic effects that they bring can never be watered down. Getting the herbal formulas right go a long way in effecting the correct treatment methods towards ascertaining the perfect healing and good health, which is the main goal of herbalism.

CHAPTER FIVE

IMPORTANT CONSIDERATIONS IN USING HERBAL MEDICINE

As much as possible, there are some things we need to look into as convincing factors that should always back our decision to use herbal medicine. If you are a lover of herbal medicine like myself, I believe you need to ask yourself some questions in line with your choice of interest. Questions like: how well do I know these herbs? Am I confident enough to convince someone skeptical about the use of herbs into being a lover of herbal medicine? How can I use herbal medicine to make a change in my community? If you can provide answers to these questions, then I believe you are good to go.

To those of that are yet to provide answers to those questions, I believe by the time you have reached this section of the book, your confidence level should have increased. And you are just a few steps away to make a significant impact on your world. To help further on this journey, I have outlined some points that discussed more on the importance of herbal medicine for our continuous use here in this section. When you know the importance of a thing, you do not need anyone to convince you further before you decide to go ahead and explore it. And even enlighten other people on what you have discovered and sure about.

Whenever you are making considerations about using herbal medicine, let the outlined points below convince you further in making what I call the right choice:

- **Soothing application to wounds:** Herbs like black pepper, cinnamon, myrrh, aloe, sandalwood, ginseng, red clover, burdock, bayberry, and safflower are used to heal wounds, sores, and boils.

- **Beautification of your environment:** Apart from the therapeutic significance of medicinal herbs, you can always plant them in your surrounding for beautification. Herbs like Basil, Fennel, Chives, Cilantro, Apple Mint, Thyme, Golden Oregano, Variegated Lemon Balm, Rosemary, and Variegated

Sage are essential medicinal herbs that can be planted in the kitchen garden. These herbs are easy to grow, look good, taste and smell amazing, and many of them are magnets for bees and butterflies.

- **Blood Purification:** Many herbs are used as blood purifiers to alter or change a long-standing condition by eliminating the metabolic toxins. These herbs are also known as 'blood cleansers.' Certain herbs improve the immunity of the person, thereby reducing diseases such as fever.

- **Antibiotics Effects:** Some herbs also have antibiotic properties. Turmeric is useful in inhibiting the growth of germs, harmful microbes, and bacteria. Turmeric is widely used as a home remedy to heal cut and wounds.

- **Antacid Effects:** Some herbs are used to neutralize the acid produced by the stomach. Examples include herbs like marshmallow root and leaf. These herbs serve as antacids, and they retain the healthy gastric acid needed for proper digestion.

- **Antidote Effects:** Indian sages were known to have remedies from plants which act against poisons from animals and snake bites.

- **Appetizers:** Herbs like Cardamom and Coriander are renowned for their appetizing qualities. Other aromatic herbs such as peppermint, cloves, and turmeric add a pleasant aroma to the food, thereby increasing the taste of the meal.

- **High Antiseptic Value:** Some herbs like aloe, sandalwood, turmeric, sheetraj hindi, and khare khasak are commonly used as antiseptic and are very high in their medicinal values.

- **Expectorants**: Ginger and cloves are used in certain cough syrups. They are known for their expectorant property, which promotes the thinning and ejection of mucus from the lungs, trachea, and bronchi. Eucalyptus, Cardamom, Wild cherry, and cloves are also expectorants.

- **Soothing Effects:** Herbal medicine practitioners recommend calmative herbs, which provide a soothing effect on the body. They are often used as sedatives.

- **Detoxifying Properties:** Certain aromatic plants such as Aloe, Goldenseal, Barberry, and Chirayata are used as mild tonics. The bitter taste of such plants reduces toxins in the blood. They help destroy infection as well.

- **Cardiac Stimulants:** Herbs such as Chamomile, Calamus, Ajwain, Basil, Cardamom, Chrysanthemum, Coriander, Fennel, Peppermint and Spearmint, Cinnamon, Ginger, and Turmeric help promote good blood circulation. Therefore, they are used as cardiac stimulants.

- **Organ Stimulants:** Certain herbs are used as stimulants to increase the activity of a system or an organ. Examples include herbs like Cayenne (Lal Mirch, Myrrh, Camphor, and Guggul.

- **Disinfectants:** There are some medicinal herbs with the disinfectant property. These properties destroy disease-causing germs. They also inhibit the growth of pathogenic microbes that cause infectious diseases.

- **Health Rejuvenation:** A wide variety of herbs, including Giloe, Goldenseal, Aloe, and Barberry are used as tonics. They can also be nutritive, and they rejuvenate human health, as well as individuals with one form of disease or the other.

- **Astringents:** Sandalwood and Cinnamon are great astringents apart from being aromatic. Sandalwood is mostly used in arresting the discharge of blood, mucus, etc.

- **Treatment of Wounds:** Honey, turmeric, marshmallow, and licorice can effectively treat a fresh cut and wound. They are termed as vulnerary herbs.

- **Temperature Balance and Anti-fever:** To reduce fever, and traditional Indian medicine practitioners recommend the production of heat caused by the condition, certain antipyretic herbs such as Chirayta, black pepper, sandal wood and safflower.

CONCLUSION

The evolution of the world around us has always been bringing dynamism to our ways of life. The technological advancement era that we are presently in one way or the other affecting lifestyle. The techno-savvy lifestyle that we have embraced is taking us away from nature. The truth is we cannot escape from nature because we are part of nature. We need to accept the fact that herbs are natural products that we have all around us. They are free from side effects. They are comparatively safe, eco-friendly, and locally available. Traditionally, there are a lot of herbs used for the ailments related to different seasons. There is a need to promote them and embrace the use of these herbs to save human lives.

Today, these herbal products are the symbol of safety in contrast to the synthetic drugs that are all around our pharmaceutical stores, which are regarded as unsafe to human being and the environment. Although herbs had been prized for their medicinal, flavoring, and aromatic qualities for centuries, the synthetic products of the modern age surpassed their importance, for a while. However, the blind dependence on synthetics is over. People are returning to the naturals with the hope of safety and security. So, let us not waste away the gift of nature, which are these herbs. Now is the time for us to enjoy the great importance that comes with these herbs and also be proud to promote them globally. Always have it in mind that *"Health is Wealth."* You have everything that it takes to live a healthy life around you. Make good use of it!

CPSIA information can be obtained
at www.ICGtesting.com
Printed in the USA
LVHW041340210621
690761LV00018B/788

9 781695 439443